A

Little

Book

About

A

BIG

Topic:

CANCER

Life ~ Living ~ Inspire

by

Carolyn Snyder

ACKNOWLEDGEMENTS

There is no real order to this love letter.

You will see how blessed I am by the people in my life.

First, my Editor and Friend

Chris Cimino

He was the first person to see my musings

and said 'I don't know what they are exactly.

But they should be seen'

And behold those musings became this book.

Thank you, Chris

You came into my life at the

Perfect time.

You have been the best combination

of

Editor, adviser

with

Humor and kindness.

It could not get better.

Angie Hanson

Angie's dedication to do Zimbaté

with me every day

has been a True Gift

of Love.

From my first surgery,

She drove to my house

Every day to work with me.

That is remarkable.

She is empathic,

Nonjudgmental.

She is a natural with Zimbaté

And continues to bless me with her presence.

She has become a dear friend.

We continue to work several times a week.

To the Village

that makes up my

Life.

The talks, the actions

The love and caring

Each person has given

In their own way.

It is your giving and

Prayers that help in a big way

To keep me on track.

~

My Family

As always, they are the Backbone

of my continuing success

With this illness.

I get daily

Phone calls and texts,

Personal attention and time

When I need it.

I love each of them Dearly.

They make my

Heart Happy.

My English Family

They come to visit.

Call often.

They all are Amazing people

and brilliant Friends.

My dearest wish

is to travel to the UK again.

The support they have given me in

My Zimbaté work and in my personal

Life has been without question the most

Lovely gift of love I have been given.

I am humbled.

To my new second Family

Wow, you blow me away.

It is an honor to be included and cared for

With such gentle kindness.

I feel loved and am doing better for

Your willing involvement.

Thank you

The Staff at SWEDISH MEDICAL CENTER

They work hard on my behalf.

I am grateful to my excellent doctors,

Jeff Ward and Tom Jurich.

The Oncology nurses are

A far step above excellence,

With knowledge,

Kindness

Humor

and Professionalism.

The nurses on Floor 8

(The only floor I ever want to be on!)

They are the very best.

I received excellent care

And felt they saw me as a Person.

Thanks to each of you.

DEDICATION

To assist those who have

Difficult situations

Or

Just may want

A new perspective

On their life circumstances.

May you find a new Twist

On an old situation

Or

A new frame for a

Fresh view of Life.

MY WISH

This little book

Was written with the

Intent

To

Encourage,

Bring awareness,

Reassure.

To help you feel understood

And cared for.

You certainly are

Not

Alone

In your journey.

Our paths through Cancer

May look different.

But they are more alike

Than unalike.

Blessings to each of You

on your Journey.

With love,

Carolyn

MY INTENT

Intent is the base

Of living.

Intent determines how

You live your life.

Clear

Positive

Intent

Will go a long way

Towards a balanced

Well-adjusted

Life.

My intent with this book

Has been clear from the

First word.

I wish to encourage,

Share my experiences,

Bring hope, and confidence

To your life experience.

You need not have Cancer

To

Receive value

From this book.

This is about living a Full

and

Productive

Life

with Joy,

Compassion,

and

Love.

Love of self and

Others.

With gratitude for life

For its surprises

and

Rich experiences.

Namasté

WHO IS THIS BOOK FOR?

Anyone who has a serious illness,

Cares for someone

With a serious situation,

Or

Has difficulties

In their own life.

Anyone

Who is interested in a

New perspective

On life and Living.

I hope there is some

Bit

That brings a light bulb

Moment,

that brings Peace,

An inner calmness

And worthiness.

We are all important

In our own special and

Unique ways.

Value yourself

Each day.

FEELINGS

I

Do not have Cancer.

I

Live *in* my body but

I

Am not *of* my body.

My body serves a purpose

Directed by me.

I am grateful.

LOVE

The human body is

Created in unique ways,

Different for every Spirit

That chooses to take a body.

Often that body is asked to

Struggle,

Hurt,

And sacrifice,

All in support of the Spirit's

Desire for knowledge,

Growth and understanding.

My body accepted that my Spirit self

Desired to experience Cancer.

It did this to assist myself and others.

We have, and will continue, to benefit greatly.

I am humbled.

WORDS

When we hear the word Cancer we want to run

Far and fast.

Fear and anger are two of the most common

Feelings.

What if I told you - *you* choose to have Cancer

To learn and grow on your own

Spiritual path?

Negative feelings are exhausting and drain

Your needed

Healing energy.

Focus on what you can learn from Cancer

And

How you can manage the everyday tasks.

You will be surprised at how many people will come forth

If you ask.

Asking can be hard.

Try it anyway.

GIFTS

When we hear the word Cancer

We put a cap on the C

And Fear in our hearts.

Yes, Cancer can be very serious.

But

The Universe is all about Balance.

Cancer gives the most amazing

Gifts.

Look past the fear and pain

And

See the beautiful, surprising,

Love and generosity

Available.

Cancer is not the enemy

THE CARING OF CANCER

What Cancer

isn't......

It is Not the boss of me.

I do Not belong to it.

Yes, it was invited into my body.

But it must improve its manners.

I will Not let it rule my life

Or

Determine what each day is made of.

I get that it has meaning for me

And

A role to play.

If

We are to coexist,

An understanding must occur.

Don't wash away my joy in my life.

Don't let me focus just on Cancer

I want to continue to play a part in others' lives,

To have fun,

To chew gum,

To be silly and not too bright.

Please, don't try to extinguish

My light.

ONCOLOGY

It is a Monday

And

I am on my way to chemo.

I look forward to going.

Strange?

Maybe....

But what I see there is that

Everyone is genuinely

Knowledgeable,

Sincere,

Kind,

Approachable.

When I am there I feel like

I am

Cared about and

My Illness matters

No!

My good health matters!

They are totally present and on my team.

I am grateful.

DOCTORS

One of the most important

Decisions...

Choosing your Doctor(s).

For me, they need

To be

Smart

and

Compassionate.

To *see me.*

Able to listen

(Really listen).

Explain easily what I don't understand.

Consider all sides of the situations.

Be honest.

Have integrity.

I would like to introduce my Doctors

Dr. Tom Jurich, surgeon

Dr. Jeff Ward, Oncology

I have been so honored

To know and work with

Two fine men and Doctors.

I am blessed

FAITH OR FEAR

When faced with

One of life's

Big moments

Where do you go?

Panic?

Fear?

Anger?

Or maybe you look Deep within yourself

To find

Faith

Strength

Love of self.

It is impossible to have

Faith and fear

At the same time.

You are at choice.

HAVE OR HAVE NOT

Do I have Cancer?

Or

Does Cancer have me?

Does cancer have you in its grip?

Do you identify it as yours?

As *My* Cancer?

Has it become part of who you are?

Do you own it?

My thinking, Cancer is a visitor

I will treat it with respect.

But I don't want to invite it

To be the boss and give it

Ownership of my Being.

I will take responsibility for Cancer's

Presence in my life.

Being very present with your body's

Needs is paramount to becoming healthy.

Food, sleep, activities, relationships

They all contribute.

Finding doctors that you trust and

And feel they see you as a

Whole person.

Cancer can be a temporary messenger.

Get the message,

Treat it with deference,

Learn what it has to offer,

Release it.

Love your body for how it tries

To protect you

Its intent is never to bring you harm

But to safeguard.

LOVING......

It is hard sometimes

To know when to Love

And

When to withdraw.

Not to withdraw Love

But

To withdraw from interaction.

Some things we need to do on our

Own.

Pain and suffering can close us off from others.

It can be most difficult to show others

Our hurt and insecurities.

We forget that not only is it rewarding to give

But hardest of all can be the ability to receive

Gracefully.

Think of the person on the other side - how thrilled they

are to give to you.

It is a way you can bring Joy to another.

Some things need to be done on our own.

Most often, things shared

Grow and

Bloom

HAIR

My hair

I look at it and I despair.

No longer full

And

Easy to style,

It is limp

And

Has lost its curl.

The chemo has done it worst...

Wait...

What exactly does it mean?

To have my hair change?

Recognizing this change means to

See

Deeper into my Being,

Past the surface of life

And

My physical, outward

Appearance.

Do I like my hair's change?

No!

But

I refuse to allow it to rule

Even

A minute of what I do with

My life.

Seeing friends,

Going to dinner,

Laughing out loud.

It is what it is.

It has no control.

But I do.

Lise #1

One morning her hair

Needed to be cut.

Ouch, that was hard.

Next came

The pain.

More hair had to go.

Her husband gently shaved her

Head.

And then

His own.

The tears flowed fast.

But

That part didn't last.

Hats

Entered her world.

All kinds.

She sported new styles,

Reinvented

Her look.

Her friends looked forward

To each new

Addition.

Each hat showed the world

Her strength,

Her ability to adjust

And

Adapt.

OWNING VS RENTING

Do I own *things?*

Or

Do they Own me?

How much do the material possessions

Rule

My world?

Do I secretly covet my friend's

New outfit?

Car?

Cancer has a way about it.

Values can change

In a flash.

With an opportunity to shop

Or

Spend time with my Daughter,

There is no

Question.

Listening to gossip

Holds no appeal.

Forgiveness comes

More easily.

Expressions of

Love

Flow.

Appreciation is

At the forefront of your

Thoughts.

Gratitude

Is a living part of each Day.

Are things a part of my life?

Yes.

But they are here for time with me

And

I can easily pass them on and

Move on to what is next.

Spend some time sorting through

Your things.

Dispose

Of what no longer has meaning.

Amazing how light and freeing

You will

Feel.

Oh, one more thing

Giving of my belongings;

To someone who

Admires them

Brings true Joy

To my heart.

LABELS

We assign meaning to everything.

Not a bad thing

Unless it affects you in a

Negative way.

When you hear the word

Chemotherapy

What is the first word that comes to mind?

Dying?

Poison?

Toxic?

Our thoughts have *great* influence

And Power.

While we make our way through

Cancer,

Are those the words you want to work with?

We actually have Chemo treatments

To get well.

I propose that we change our

Thinking.

Chemo is there to get rid of

Cancer cells.

I believe that we can lessen

The effect of Chemo on

Normal cells

By our thinking,

How we talk about it,

How we feel about Chemo.

If we are grateful for the chance to

Get well,

Thank Chemo,

Bless the process.

And

KNOW

We are not harmed

By our treatments.

Who knows what can be accomplished?

Does this sound too fanciful?

Does that even matter?

Live on the wild side

Experiment

See how Powerful

You can be.

You will amaze yourself!

Lise #2

Going out in public

With

No hair,

Body a new shape,

People's eyes on her.

What will they think?

Well,

Who cares?!

She dresses with care,

Puts on subtle makeup,

No hat.

Let's make a statement!

Meeting her Mother and Sister

at the Opera House,

Lise was elegant,

Beautiful,

Stunning,

As only a woman

Who has

Confidence in

Who she is,

Loves herself,

And is willing to share

With the world

Can be.

What an impactful,

Lovely gift of

Herself

To share with the

World.

GOALS

(Commonly known

As a bucket list.)

One of my motivations

To stay

Healthy, active, positive

Are nifty adventures

To look forward to.

So here is a sneak preview.

French Laundry or Masa's in NYC.

A cruise, especially a river boat in Europe.

Hawaii.

Bryce Canyon.

Back to Orcas House.

Own a Mini car.

There are more but these are some of the

Special ones.

Will I be able to do them?

Can I even afford them?

Don't know and don't care.

Having them available,

I will find a way

If the opportunity presents

Itself.

MOTIVATION

My bucket list is filled mostly with

Big activities.

The bigger question is

How to stay

Mentally and Emotionally up

On the daily

Struggle?

There so many little things that can make you

Feel joy,

Accomplished,

Satisfied and Fulfilled.

Clean a closet, a drawer.

Have special food treat.

Be with friends.

Go to a new place for lunch.

The beach (you do need water for this one!).

To a movie, an art show.

Knit (I'm getting better!).

Paint a picture (afraid I am not getting better!).

You get my drift.

You need to make a plan.

Don't fill your days with just activities.

You need lots of quiet time,

Alone time to be a blank slate,

Think thought and listen.

Get creative.

Make fun.

Make happy.

Even if it is seeing a lovely (fill in the blank),

It is another challenge.

Are you up for it?

MORE...

I got up this AM and found I have more to say

About Motivation.

One of the areas is your personal look.

On really hard days I don't do anything but

Jammies, no fussing with

Hair or makeup - and I don't go out in the world!

After a couple of days

Cleaning up,

Putting on something I like,

Fixing my hair, a little makeup,

And I actually feel better.

How you see Yourself is

Important.

Get your hair cut, try a new style,

Try red streaks.

Be adventuresome.

Do your nails.

Buy some lotion that makes you

Smile when you put it on.

Another very good remedy?

Do something for someone else.

Call and tell them how important

They are to you.

Send a card.

Bake cookies.

Do that same thing for someone else

That brings joy to you.

The reward for you is a

Worthy endeavor well done.

This will assist others in their

Healing and health.

Happiness and that bubble of Joy

Is such a gift.

WHO IS GOING TO BE RESPONSIBLE?

What a dilemma!

My body has this Cancer,

And

Who is going to be accountable for

All the choices?

Me? NO, I have enough going on

Just

Having Cancer in my body.

I know, my Doctor, which would be good.

My Daughter, she can make all the decisions.

She loves me.

Or

My best friend, she is a good manager and smart.

What a relief, I will just do what they

Tell me to do.

STOP!

Alert!

Do I want others to shoulder

My life choices?

How painful for them

To bear the burdens of another?

This is my life.

I need to have the guts to Live it,

Trust myself to do what needs to be done -

For Me.

RESPONSIBILITY

Cancer is one of the Big Ones

In life.

If you take responsibility,

It is an empowering gift you

Give to yourself.

No,

Don't do it alone

Seek advice from those that you

Trust

And

Listen

To what they say.

But you need to make the final

Decisions.

PAYING ATTENTION

For me, in May, my scans showed

No tumors...

To continue with chemo?

To stop chemo?

My concerns?

Yes, Cancer could come back.

I had done an 18 month marathon

Which included

Two major abdominal surgeries and

Continuing chemo.

No chance for my body to heal from any of that.

And I didn't go into this healthy.

I wanted to stop all treatment and regroup.

I presented my side of the issues to

Everyone I trusted.

Almost everyone wanted me to continue

Treatments.

They also said they would support

Whatever my decision was going to be.

I declined more treatments.

I spent the next 2 ½ months

Enjoying summer, getting healthy

And having fun!

Four tumors showed up the 1st of August

No question, back to chemo.

I am in my third cycle of this series.

I am handling

Chemo better.

My body is Stronger.

I am mentally Stronger.

Did I make the best decision?

For me, I did.

Was it hard to go against others'

Opinions?

Yes.

Very.

I am blessed that my decision didn't

Change any of my relationships.

I knew that my body needed to recharge.

So,

I listened.

At this time, that was the right choice

For Me.

Next big decision?

I will continue to listen to others

And myself.

TRUST

Have Faith that whatever

Comes up, you will have the Ability

To meet the challenges.

Take a chance that you have the Tools

To live your life,

And

Love yourself

with Grace.

OSTOMY TALE

At my second surgery

I received an

Ostomy bag.

They could not get all of

Tumors

And needed to place

An ostomy bag

On my abdomen.

I was not conscious much on the First

Day

My friend told me that I was

Not pleased.

At all.

Well, on the Second Day after Surgery,

I didn't really have an

Opinion.

It was just there.

A little odd, but

Oh, well!

I had a wonderful Home Nurse

Who showed me the

Ropes,

The care of my new part.

At first it took 45 minutes to

Change my bag.

Now I can do it in minutes.

The same for emptying

My bag.

It is all pretty easy *peasy*.

The interesting part?

It is not Icky,

Disgusting,

Revolting,

The list could on.

Without that bag

I would not be alive!

I can only be grateful for

My Doctor, who did a

Splendid job.

Yes, there are people who

Can't handle my ostomy

And

Their first question,

Can it be reversed?

I have no idea.

I have bigger

Things to focus on.

It will not matter one

Way or the other.

If you are having a difficult time

Adjusting,

Email me.

Life totally goes on

I even swim!

In the big picture of

Cancer,

This is a small issue.

And really don't let it

Rule your life or have

Control over You.

After all,

You

Are the Boss.

DYING

When faced with the idea of dying

I wanted to ask for help.

What does one *do?*

Run around franticly, doing what for whom?

Clean house, write letters, take trips, and cry?

Feel guilty for reading a book or watching a TV
program?

There is no magical manual.

But wait....

There is Magic.

A very quiet, soft guidance.

Slowly I realized that there was a difference within me.

My heart opened more and I found that being fully
Present

Was *easier*.

I was *freer*.

I didn't hold back my praise and love.

I take each moment as it comes.

My Appreciation for those around me runs deep

And I have been sharing my Gratitude.

The Nurses were endlessly kind

And

Have taken such good care of me.

My family and friends seem to know what to say and

When to say it.

I know when I depart - where I will be going and I look forward to

Home.

I still have things to do here; I may or may not get them done.

But I feel good about My life.

It has not changed all that much from before Cancer

But it has

Greater depth,

A peace,

Understanding and a Willingness to Give.

Appreciation

And so much

Gratitude.

DEPARTURE

I feel like I will

Depart

This Earth

When I have done what I

Set out to do.

Not any earlier

Nor later.

The timing will be

Perfect.

I will not die.

Because

When I depart, that will

Not be my ending.

Did you know that

There is

One breathe

Between

Being of this Earth

And

Moving on to our next

Experience?

Pretty amazing

This life.

SUPPORT

Why is it important

That someone is *willing* to

Hear it all?

The good, the bad,

And the ugly.

The highs,

The *aha* moments,

The gifts

Cancer gives

You.

It is the sharing of love,

Real love,

Real compassion,

Real understanding.

This is a gift beyond

My ability to express

Properly.

Which holds my

Unending

Appreciation, admiration,

And love.

Everyone needs someone like

You.

Aren't I the Lucky one!

INTUITION

Call it what you may

Hunch,

Sixth Sense,

Gut Reaction,

Or the little quiet

Voice.

What is important is that

You add it to your

Toolbox of tricks.

With all the decisions

To make,

Paths to take.

Every little bit help.

And this is a Major

Participant.

Actually, *intuition* is a

Key to Living life

With greater ease and

Less fumbles.

Tonight my Brother called

And suggested that

I try

Hypnosis.

I got this big 'hit' that said

YES!

So, tomorrow I will give

A call and

See where this takes me.

I am excited.

Thanks, Jim

FRIENDS

What defines

Friendship?

It can vary from

Friend to Friend.

What I do know about

Friendship

Is that it is

Precious,

Needs to be

Nurtured,

Loved,

And

Treasured.

Each Friend brings something

Different,

Will meet different needs

You have.

Please remember!

Although your needs seem

Huge and overwhelming,

Your Friend will need *your* attention

At times.

Friendships are a two-way

Street.

Keep active in others' lives,

It is healthy and will make you

Happy to give to

Another.

Love you, Rachael!

GRATITUDE

Expressing gratitude

Daily

Is one of the tools that each of us

Should use,

When we are ill or well.

Going to the place that holds

Gratitude,

Finding that something

That warms your Heart,

Then

Bring it forth into the light.

I have a Friend.

We share our Gratitude

Each day

With each other.

We don't comment.

We just Share.

It sets up the day so nicely.

It makes me aware that

Regardless of my circumstances

There is always

Time and room

In my life

For

Gratitude.

It can change

Your whole

Day.

Or

Your whole life.

TRUTH

What is Truth

To you?

Does your truth come

Without malice?

Or ego?

For me, my illness, has made me aware

That telling the Truth,

Being Honest,

Is freeing

And loving.

What I find in my relationships is

The desire

To

Let people know I

Appreciate them,

Love them.

When I think to compliment,

I do.

I give my honest opinions.

But I am careful to be

Kind.

Illness does not give you the right to

Blast through the

Heart of someone else

And

Wound them.

But it does give you the right to express

Your thoughts.

When you inwardly watch your

Reactions and emotions,

And act with care,

There can be a bubble of joy

That sits right over your heart.

It is a

Lovely thing to experience!

CONTROL

Okay, you have Cancer.

Rest, Exercise and

Nutrition.

These three are in your control.

Or are they?

It is a delicate balance.

Some days I am so tired that

A nap starts at 10:00 AM and

And continues until 3:00 PM.

Exercise is the same.

The Idea of exercise does me in some days.

Mostly I do it.

And mostly it is a benefit.

But, there is the day

When it is too much for

My body and I overdo.

I am good about sleep at night

And I am learning to rest during the day.

FOOD

Food is another issue that

Stumps me.

Often nothing looks good and I end up throwing food away.

So, do I eat and hope to derive some

Pleasure and Value

From my choice?

YES!!

I do not often eat balanced meals.

I always drink Ensure®, at least twice a day.

It brings nutritional balance.

On the days I can't get anything down?

Ice cream, cottage cheese,

Cold foods work well.

Well into the second week of chemo

My appetite can come back with a vengeance!

I want to eat everything in sight

And

Pretty much do!

At first, I was slightly obsessed with

How much of this and how long to do that.

I found it exhausting.

Much too stiff to manage.

I have relaxed.

I know what is good for me.

Do I always do it?

No.

I have found that my blood draws show my nutritional

Levels are normal and stable.

They show flexibility - even when I don't!

What do I want to say about all this?

Relax!

Every little thing will not make a difference,

Except to your mental and emotional health.

Love and laugh, and

Live.

With

Gratitude.

A PATH

Each of us has our Own

Path.

We have no way of knowing

The purpose

Of someone's

Path.

The dirty street person

May be a beautiful

Soul

Wanting the specific

Experience of being

Shunned,

Avoided

With no eyes seeing *him.*

Just his surface exterior.

The person with

Cancer

May wants you to see

The person behind the

Cancer.

Those of us with Cancer

Fight

the Good Fight with a

Disease, but also the

Stigma associated

With Cancer.

Who knows why I have Cancer?

Do you?

Does it really matter what is

Going on in our

Bodies?

Look past

The cover we present

To the Essence

And to the

Heart.

People in crisis often have opened

To Great Truths and

Have wisdom beyond

Understanding.

Open yourself and see the

Those around you with

New eyes

And

An open heart.

MY SECRET WEAPON

I do a form of hands on healing

Called

Zimbaté

(Pronounced *zim-ba-tay*)

It is for mind, body, and spirit

To heal yourself, to make positive changes in

Your life.

To know your Path.

For me

It has lessened the side effects of chemo,

Helped heal the tumors,

Keeping my body in Balance

My mental state - stable

My emotional state – healthy.

I am grateful every day to have such a gift

In my toolbox.

If something like this is attractive to you

Give it try.

THANK YOU

I hope that you have received

Value,

Information

And

A tickle of interest in

Some of the concepts

From this little book.

May your life journey be

Sweeter,

Kinder,

More

Empathic

for Yourself and others.

Appreciate *your* journey.

It is not always easy.

But it can also

Have amazing rewards

With a great sense of gratitude

For being able to share

Myself with you.

Thank you.

I wish to share some of the quotes

That have made an impact or influenced my life.

They came into my life at 'just the right' time.

I am sure that you have your own

Stash of words that have meaning for you.

Enjoy and may they bring you joy.

Carolyn

THE PATH

Watch your thoughts;

They become words.

Watch your words;

They become actions.

Watch your actions;

They become habits.

Watch your habits;

They become character.

Watch your character;

It becomes destiny.

Anonymous

Everything is energy and that is all there is to it.
Match the frequency of the reality you want and you cannot help but get what you want.
It can be no other way.
This is not philosophy,
This is physics.

Albert Einstein

In the end, only three things matter:

How much you loved,

How gently you lived,

And how gracefully you let go of the

Things not meant for you.

Buddha

~ One of my goals for this lifetime ~

To get out of

My own way

Carolyn

The best way to find yourself

is to lose yourself in the

Service of others

Gandhi

We all worship.

We choose what it is we will worship

Unknown

Who am I?

Nothing real can be threatened.

Nothing unreal exists

Herein lies the Peace of

God.

Dr. Helen Schucman,
A Course in Miracles

People often say that this or that person

Has not yet found himself.

The self is not something you find,

It is something one creates

Thomas Szasz

Experience

Reading a book

Knowledge

What you learn from a book

(Where most people stop)

Wisdom

Being able to apply it your life

Understanding

Integration of the wisdom into your life

Guidance

Using the wisdom to help others

Unknown

When you give up everything, you will get everything you need.

Anonymous

A true friend is someone who reaches for your hand and touches your heart.

Antoine de Saint-Exupery

Don't let a little dispute injure a great friendship

Remember the three R's Respect for self, Respect for others: and Responsibility for all your actions.

Your truth sits in your heart
When you lose, don't lose the lesson
Learn the rules so you know how to break them properly
Remember, that not getting what you want is sometimes a wonderful stroke of luck.
Great love and great achievements involve great risk

Dalai Lama

EGO   Earth Guidance Only

Understanding Your Existence

FAITH

When you have come to the edge of all the light you

know, and are about to step off in the darkness of the

unknown, Faith is knowing one of two things will

happen: There will be something solid to stand on or

you will be taught how to fly.

Patrick Overton